When Hearing Loss *Ambushes Your Ears*

Here's What Happens When Your Hearing Goes on the Fritz

Second Edition

Neil G. Bauman, Ph.D.

Integrity First Publications

Lynden, WA   http://IntegrityFirstPublications.com

When Hearing Loss Ambushes Your Ears
Here's What Happens When Your Hearing Goes on the Fritz

Second Edition

Another **Integrity First** book in the series:

Everything You Wanted to Know About Your Hearing Loss But Were Afraid to Ask (Because You Knew You Wouldn't Hear the Answers Anyway!)

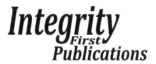

Integrity *First* **Publications**

1013 Ridgeway Drive,
Lynden, WA 98264-1057
Phone: (360) 778-1266
FAX: (360) 389-5226
Email: info@IntegrityFirstPublications.com
Website: http://IntegrityFirstPublications.com

Printed in the United States of America

Warning—Disclaimer

This book is for your education and reference. It is neither a medical manual nor a guide to self-treatment for medical problems. Do not construe this book as giving personal medical advice or instruction. The author is not a medical doctor and neither prescribes treatment nor treats medical problems and does not intend that you attempt to do so either. If you suspect that you have a medical problem related to your ears, seek competent professional medical help. Use the information in this book to help you make informed decisions, not as a substitute for any treatment that your doctor may have prescribed for you.

The information and opinions expressed in this book are the result of careful research. They are believed to be accurate and sound, based on the best judgment available to the author. If you fail to consult appropriate health professionals, you assume the risk of any injuries. Neither Integrity First Publications, the Center for Hearing Loss Help, nor the author assumes any responsibility for damages or losses incurred as a result of using the information in this book, nor for any errors or omissions. It is the responsibility of each reader to exercise good judgment in using any information contained in this book.

Contents

About the Author

Neil G. Bauman, Ph.D., (Dr. Neil), is the C.E.O. of the Center for Hearing Loss Help. He is a hearing loss coping skills specialist, researcher, author and speaker on issues pertaining to hearing loss. No stranger to hearing loss himself, he has lived with a life-long, severe, hereditary hearing loss.

Dr. Neil did not let his hearing loss stop him from achieving what he wanted to do. He earned several degrees in fields ranging from forestry to ancient astronomy (Ph. D.) and theology (Th. D.) in addition to his extensive studies in fields related to hearing loss.

His mission is helping hard of hearing people understand and successfully cope with their hearing losses and other ear conditions. To this end, he provides education, support and counsel to hard of hearing people through personal contact, as well as through his books, articles, presentations and seminars.

Dr. Neil is the author of eleven books and more than 1,000 articles on hearing-loss related topics. (See the back of this book for a list of his books.) In addition, he is a dynamic speaker. His presentations are in demand throughout the USA and Canada.

He is a member of the Hearing Loss Association of America and the Canadian Hard of Hearing Association.

You can reach him at:

Neil Bauman, Ph.D.
Center for Hearing Loss Help
1013 Ridgeway Drive
Lynden, WA 98264-1057
Phone: (360) 778-1266
FAX: (260) 389-5226
Email: neil@hearinglosshelp.com
Web site: http://hearinglosshelp.com

Chapter 1

What's Happening to My Hearing?

You know that your hearing isn't what it used to be. Maybe it changed all of a sudden. You wonder, "What's going wrong with my ears? Is my hearing going to get worse? Am I going deaf? Is there anything I can do about it? Are there any operations that will help me?"

You are right to be concerned about your hearing. And yes, there are many things you can do to help yourself. First, however, you need to know more about how your ears work and what is changing. Then you will be far better equipped to help yourself.

Our Marvelous Ears and How They Work

Our ears are incredible hearing organs. They are masterpieces of ingenuity, securely nestled deep in our skulls. They are extremely sensitive yet reasonably robust. For example, the softest sound people with normal hearing typically hear is 0 decibels (dB). Somewhere around 110 dB sounds get to be painfully loud, but we can still readily understand them. Is this sound just 110 times louder? Most definitely not! Since the decibel scale is logarithmic, a sound of 110 dB takes **100 billion times** more sound energy to produce than a sound of 0 dB. Unbelievably, our ears can hear this tremendously loud sound without damage (if it is just for a few minutes or less). No wonder David exclaimed, "I will praise you [God]; for I am fearfully and wonderfully made: marvelous are Your works; and that my soul knows right well".[1]

Full Size Already?

Did you know that when you were born the three miniature bones in each of your middle ears were already full size?

Human ears consist of three parts—the outer ear, middle ear and inner ear (Fig. 1-1). Here is how they work.

The **outer ear** is the only part of our ears that we can actually see. (Doctors call it the pinna or auricle.) Our pinnae collect the sound waves from the air and funnel them into our inch (or inch and a half) long ear canals. Our ear canals do two things. First, they protect our delicate eardrums from damage. Second, they resonate certain frequencies of sound that are necessary for understanding speech. This makes these sounds louder and easier to hear before they even reach our eardrums.

Our ear canals end at our eardrums. (The fancy medical term for eardrum is "tympanic membrane"). Eardrums are semi-transparent, pearly-grey, strong, yet tissue-paper thin skin membranes stretched tightly across the inner end of our ear canals. They consist of three layers of tissue—skin on the outside,

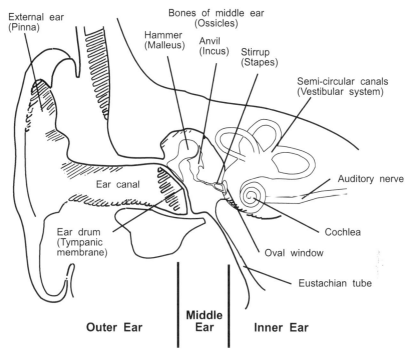

Fig. 1-1. A cross section of the auditory system showing the various parts of the outer, middle and inner ear.

connective tissue to make them taut and stiff in the middle, and a mucus membrane on the inside.

We likely think of our eardrums as flat round disks, but they are really concave—their centers point inward—much like loudspeaker cones.[2]

Eardrums change the sound waves that hit them into mechanical vibrations.

Our **middle ears** are air-filled chambers about the size of large peas. They contain three tiny bones. (Doctors call them ossicles.) These bones are the smallest bones in our bodies. Because of their distinctive shapes, we commonly call them the hammer (malleus), anvil (incus), and stirrup (stapes). These bones are actually tiny levers, hinged together. They amplify and transmit the vibrations of our

11

eardrums across our middle ears to our oval windows in the base of our cochleas (COKE-lee-ah). They do this by taking the movements of the comparatively large eardrum, compressing it and focusing it all on the minuscule foot-plate of the stirrup. The stirrup, in turn, vigorously raps on the oval window. These three tiny bones actually amplify the sounds they receive from our eardrums about 150 percent by the time the stirrup passes them to the oval window.[3]

Our middle ears not only amplify sounds, they can also reduce the volume of extra loud sounds and lower pitched sounds (commonly unwanted noise) because they also contain incredible built-in ear protectors. They do this by means of two tiny muscles. The tensor tympani is attached to the hammer and pulls it slightly away from the eardrum when a loud sound is present. Likewise, the stapedius muscle connects to the stirrup and pulls it slightly away from the oval window in response to loud sounds.

Thus, when a loud noise assaults our ears, this acoustic reflex action kicks in and reduces the sound level so there is less chance of damage to the delicate hair cells in the cochlea. However, this acoustic reflex action does not act quickly enough to completely protect our ears from sudden loud sounds such as a gun blast close to our ears.

Incidentally, this acoustic reflex action has another function you might never suspect. It also kicks in automatically when we speak to reduce the sounds of our voices so that we don't deafen ourselves when speaking![4]

A small Eustachian tube connects each middle ear to the back of our throats. These Eustachian tubes are normally closed at one end but temporarily open when we swallow, yawn, sneeze or blow our noses vigorously. This action exchanges the air in our middle ears, equalizes the air pressure and refreshes the oxygen supply to the lining of our middle ears.

Allowing the pressure in our middle ears to equalize with the outside air pressure protects our delicate ear mechanisms from damage due to changes in air pressure. If this didn't happen, our eardrums could burst from the excess pressure built up there. As we all probably know, if we don't swallow or yawn when we go up or down a long, steep hill in a car or fly in a plane, pressure builds up in our middle ears. When great enough, this pressure or the accompanying pain forces us to swallow and relieve the pressure, and we hear our ears "popping". This indicates that our Eustachian tubes have momentarily opened and equalized the air pressure.

We Hear Myriads of Sounds

The human ear can distinguish and absorb more than 350,000 different sounds. From these myriads of sounds our brains produce meaning.[5]

Our **inner ears** are about the size of cherries and consist of two parts. We use one part, the cochlea, for hearing. The other part, the vestibular system, labyrinth, or semi-circular canals gives us our sense of balance and motion.

Each cochlea looks like a small snail shell consisting of two and one half turns. It is filled with two fluids (endolymph & perilymph) and contains 27,000 to 30,000 or more tiny hair cells.[6] Each hair cell has many microscopic hairs attached to it. At the base of the cochlea is the membranous oval window.

The last bone in our middle ears, the stirrup (stapes), is attached to the outside of this oval window. When the stirrup vibrates it moves the oval window with it. Thus, the mechanical motion of the three bones of our middle ears changes into the hydraulic (or wave) motion of the fluid inside the cochlea.

The movement of the fluid in the cochlea causes the tiny hairs (cilia) to move with it, much like grass moves in the wind. The movement of these minuscule hairs stimulates the hair cells to which they are attached. They, in turn, generate tiny electrical impulses. The endings of our auditory nerves (a branch of the 8th cranial nerve) pick up these electrical impulses and send them to our brains. Our brains interpret these electrical impulses, and we then "hear" them as speech, music or noise.

Hair Cells Incredibly Sensitive

The hair cells in each cochlea are so incredibly sensitive that they will respond to cilia movements of one millionth of a millimetre (about one 25 millionth of an inch).[7] That is a movement of only 10 angstroms—the distance across 10 minuscule hydrogen atoms, a small distance indeed!

The hair cells at the base of the cochlea are sensitive to high-frequency sounds while those at the tip respond to low-frequency sounds. Extremely loud sounds cause free radicals to form in the cochlea. These free radicals then "zap" any cells they come into contact with. If a free radical mortally wounds a hair cell, it dies. Since hair cells do not regenerate, when this happens, we no longer hear the sounds associated with those hair cells.

The vestibular system is the second part of our inner ears. It comes out of the base of the cochlea. This structure gives us our sense of balance and keeps us right side up. It consists of three semi-circular canals (labyrinth) and two sac-like structures—the utricle and saccule. Much like the cochlea, these canals contain a fluid and many highly-sensitive hair cells. The cillia on the hair cells in these canals let our brains know when our bodies change position. For example, if I move my head, the fluid "sloshing" around in these canals bends the sensitive cilia on the hair cells. The hair cells then send a message to my brain telling it about my new position.[8]

Your Ears Never Sleep

Did you know that your ears never sleep? Even when you are sleeping they are alert and constantly sending information to your brain. If your brain thinks a sound is important, it will wake you up. That is why you wake up to a baby's cry or your smoke alarm or to a furtive footfall outside your bedroom window.

Types of Hearing Loss

Your hearing loss can be one of two basic types—conductive or sensorineural (sen-sore-ee-NOOR-al) Of course, you could have both types at once. We call this a mixed hearing loss.

Conductive Hearing Loss

Conductive hearing losses result from conditions that affect our ear canals, eardrums or the three bones of our middle ears. A conductive hearing loss just means that something is preventing sounds from being effectively conducted through our middle ears. The simplest kind of conductive hearing loss to fix would be wax build-up (or some other obstruction) in our ear canals partially preventing the sound from reaching our eardrums. If our eardrums are damaged, they won't transmit the sounds to the three bones of our middle ears. This is a second cause of conductive hearing loss. If we have otosclerosis (AH-toe-sklair-OH-sis) (calcium build-up on the bones of our middle ears), they are not free to move (vibrate). When this happens, they cannot pass the sounds on to our inner ears. Fluid build-up in our middle ears also gives this same result.

Doctors estimate that approximately 10 percent of all adult hearing losses are conductive.[9] However, in children conductive hearing losses account for a whopping 90 percent of all hearing losses.[10] Conductive hearing losses are usually temporary and generally respond to medical treatment.

When Hearing Loss Strikes

About 5 percent of hard of hearing people were born with a hearing loss or acquired one before they were 3 years old. Between 3 and 18 years of age another 15 percent lose part of their hearing. However, it is after age 19 that about 80 percent of all hearing losses occur.[11]

Typically, if you have a conductive hearing loss you will still hear all frequencies of sound, but the sounds you hear will not be as loud as they once were. However, if these sounds are amplified you will then still clearly understand speech. This is a major difference between conductive and sensorineural hearing losses. Amplifying sounds for those of us with sensorineural hearing losses does not necessarily increase our understanding of speech.

A person with a conductive hearing loss often speaks softly, especially in noisy situations. Also, he can usually hear quite well in noisy situations because other people raise their voices to overcome the noise that he doesn't hear as loud as they do.

If you have a conductive hearing loss, your hearing may fluctuate. This ever-changing nature of conductive hearing losses can drive you right around the bend—and everyone else around you goes along for the ride!

Hearing Loss in Students

In 1993, a survey of about 20,000 hard of hearing students in the United States revealed how they lost their hearing.[12]

Heredity	32%
Meningitis	20%
Infections/high fevers	11%
Pregnancy complications	11%
Premature birth	11%
Middle ear infections	9%
Other	6%

Sensorineural Hearing Loss

Although commonly called nerve deafness, the correct term for an inner ear hearing loss is sensorineural hearing loss. Sensorineural hearing losses stem from problems in our inner ears—the cochlea and auditory nerves. Normally, damage occurs to the hair cells in our inner ears, often from certain drugs or loud sounds. In addition to hearing loss, sensorineural losses interfere with our ability to distinguish one sound from another. About 90 per cent of adults with hearing losses have a sensorineural hearing loss.[13] Conversely, only about 10 percent of children have this type of hearing loss.

Sensorineural hearing losses are considerably more serious than conductive losses. Furthermore, they usually involve more severe hearing losses, which typically cannot be corrected either medically or surgically.

If you have a sensorineural hearing loss, you will hear speech if it is loud enough, but often you will have difficulty understanding what is being said. Just as typically, you will hear lower frequency sounds but not the higher-frequency sounds. People often will sound like they are mumbling and slurring their words.

Causes of Hearing Loss

We can lose our hearing at any time. It may occur before we are even born, or it may only come with advancing age. There are several major causes of hearing loss. These include getting older (28%), noise in general (23%), ear infections (12%), a brief loud noise (10%), ear injuries (5%), and at birth (4%).[14]

Aging. As people live longer, their chance of becoming hard of hearing from age alone increases. There is not much we can do to prevent this apart from protecting our ears from loud sounds, avoiding drugs that cause hearing loss, eating a diet that promotes good health and getting adequate exercise.

Genetic Factors. Heredity is responsible for about 40 per cent of those who are either born with a severe hearing loss or develop one at an early age.[15]

Inherited Hearing Loss

About 10 percent of those born with a hearing loss have a form of inherited hearing loss that results in half of the children (on the average) in such families having similar hearing losses. This kind of hearing loss stems from carrying a dominant gene for hearing loss, as opposed to carrying a recessive gene which on the average only affects 1 in 4 people in families that carry this gene.

Typically, in people with dominant genetic hearing losses, hearing loss affects both ears (bilateral hearing loss) and is moderate to profound (60 to 100 dB) in severity.[16]

This is the kind of hearing loss that runs in my family. My mother was the only one of four (surviving) children with a hearing loss (1/4). She had three children, two of whom have hearing losses (2/3). I am one of those. One of my two daughters has a similar hearing loss (1/2) as well as one of my brother's three children (1/3). This is more or less the 50/50 chance expected for this type of inherited hearing loss. And yes, all of us have similar hearing losses in both ears. Also, our losses are all either moderate or severe.

Middle Ear Infections (repetitive or chronic). These are, by far, the most common cause of acquired hearing losses in young children. Middle ear infections often occur following a common cold. These infections usually clear up with appropriate treatment. Continuing (chronic) middle ear infections can cause a lifetime of hearing troubles.

Excessive Noise. Today our ears are regularly bombarded by noise. The end result is hearing loss that could have (and should have) been prevented. See Chapter 3 for more on this needless waste of hearing and what you can do about it.

Certain Medications. More than 400 prescription (and other) drugs can harm our hearing. We call drugs that can damage our ears by the fancy term of ototoxic drugs. You can learn about ototoxic drugs, herbals and chemicals in my book, *Ototoxic Drugs Exposed—The Shocking Truth About Prescription Drugs, Medications, Chemicals and Herbals That Can (and Do) Damage Our Ears*. (See the back of this book for the details on obtaining this book.)

Sudden Hearing Loss

Hearing loss may occur gradually or suddenly. It may affect one ear only or both ears. Hearing loss may vary from mild to profound. Here are some of the causes of sudden hearing loss that can affect both ears at once:

Autoimmune disorders
Measles
Meningitis
Multiple sclerosis
Ototoxic drugs
Scarlet fever
Syphilis
Systemic infections
Tuberculosis
Typhoid fever

Sudden hearing loss that only affects one ear could be from such causes as:

Acoustic neuroma
Blows to the head or ear
Herpes zoster
Meniere's disease
Mumps
Membrane rupture in the inner ear
Syphilis
Vascular disorders
Viruses such as influenza[17]

Tumors. Although relatively rare, a tumor (lesion) pressing on the auditory nerve (called an acoustic neuroma)[18] can cause hearing loss.

German Measles and Other Factors. About 60 percent of children born with hearing losses have losses that come from such causes as maternal rubella (the mother catches German measles while she is pregnant), drugs taken by the mother while pregnant, and premature birth.

Preventing Hearing Loss—Here Is What You Can Do

Is there anything we can do to prevent hearing loss? In many cases there is. We could prevent a staggering amount of hearing loss if we would just do four things. First, prevent maternal rubella. Second, vigorously and completely treat all middle ear infections. Included in this is making the necessary diet and lifestyle changes to avoid getting such infections in the first place. Third, drastically reduce our use of ototoxic drugs. Finally, and this is the most important, protect our ears from any and all loud sounds and excessive noise.[19]

The message is clear: the more noise we subject our ears to today, the less we'll hear of any sounds tomorrow. Unfortunately, far too many people seem willing to accept some degree of hearing loss in the pursuit of their work or pleasure.

As Margo put it, "When driving alone, it's just fun sometimes to pull my hearing aids out and blast the radio. Here's this white-headed hard of hearing lady blasting the radio (just so she can hear it) pulling up besides these young kids blasting their radio (deliberately) going deaf. What a contrast!" And I add, "What a useless tragedy!"

Here are some other things you can do to help prevent hearing loss. Did you know that smoking, foods high in caffeine, and fatty foods can adversely affect your hearing? This is because all three reduce the blood flow to your ears and may interfere with the natural healing of the small blood vessels that may be damaged by exposure to loud sounds. In one study of 2,348 aerospace factory workers, researchers found that smokers had greater hearing loss than did non-smokers. So if you smoke, quit. If you drink coffee or colas, change to decaffeinated brews and cut your intake of fatty foods.[20] Your ears will thank you by giving you better hearing.

Furthermore, when there are higher levels of carbon monoxide or alcohol in your bloodstream (as is often the case when you are in noisy, smoky night-clubs), you are even more vulnerable to hearing loss from loud noise.[21,22] Researchers at Johns Hopkins University found that rats exposed to loud noise and the amount of carbon monoxide produced from smoking a single cigarette suffered a permanent 20 dB hearing loss after just one exposure.[23]

Chapter 3 contains important information on how you can protect your hearing when you are in noisy places.

Chapter 1 Endnotes

1   Psalm 139:14.
2   Vernick, 1993. p. 11.

3   Olsson, 1996. p. 2.
4   Moore, 1982. p. 15.
5   Himber, 1989. p. 57.
6   Himber, 1989. p. 57.
7   New Sounds Inside The Ear, 1989. p. 58.
8   Vernick, 1993. p. 18.
9   Shimon, 1992. p. 41.
10   Chartrand, 1988. p. 14.
11   Holt, 1994. p. 3.
12   Holt, 1994. p. 4.
13   Alpiner, 1987. p. 388.
14   Holt, 1994. p. 4.
15   Hardy, 1974. p. 81.
16   Hardy, 1974. p. 84.
17   Ingrao, 1996. p. 1.
18   Hardy, 1974. p. 42.
19   Hardy, 1974. p. 43.
20   Stanten, 1996. p. 16.
21   Wilson, J. 1993. p. 9.
22   Vernick, 1993. p. 41.
23   Vernick, 1993. p. 158.

Chapter 2

Understanding Your Hearing Loss

The first step in successfully coping with your hearing loss is educating yourself. You need to learn all you can about your loss. The more you know, the more comfortable and accepting you will become. As a result, you will be able to cope ever so much better with your hearing loss.

Sound Levels and What They Mean

Sound levels and hearing loss are intimately tied together. We measure both sound levels and our hearing losses in interesting units called decibels (dB). There are three things you should know about a decibel. First, a decibel is not a given intensity

---

The (deci) Bel

A decibel is one tenth of a Bel. Incidentally, the Bel was named after Alexander Graham Bell, the famous inventor of the telephone and a teacher of the deaf. Because the Bel is such a large unit of measurement, we normally use the smaller unit, decibel, when talking about sound levels.

(loudness) of sound, but a **ratio** of how many times louder (or softer) the sound is than a given reference sound level. Second, electronics technicians working with amplifiers (such as telephone amplifiers) measure the sound **intensity** using one reference level, whereas audiologists measure your hearing loss using sound **pressure** with another reference level, yet both use the decibel as their unit of measurement! Third, the decibel is not a linear unit of measurement like a foot or meter, rather it is non-linear unit that involves logarithms.

> **Measuring Sound Levels**
>
> A sound level meter measures the pressure of sounds. When measuring sound levels, set the sound meter to the "A" scale—the scale which most closely matches the sounds human ears hear[1] and set the fast/slow response switch to slow response.

This means that 0 dB is not the absence of sound, but is an arbitrary zero. It is defined as the faintest sound that a young sensitive human ear can hear. Furthermore, because the dB scale is logarithmic, a sound intensity of 20 dB is not twice as loud as a sound intensity of 10 dB, but is 10 times as loud, and a sound intensity of 30 dB is 100 times as loud as a sound intensity of 10 dB.

The threshold of human hearing is 0 dB. At the high end, a jet plane makes a sound of about 140 dB about 100 feet from the engine. This is painful and will quickly and permanently damage your hearing. At 170 dB, sound can literally blow you off your feet.[2]

This brief look at how we measure sounds will help you to understand how we classify hearing loss.

Perceived Loudness vs. Actual Loudness

For roughly every 10 dB increase in sound intensity, we perceive the sound as being twice as loud, when in actual fact, the sound intensity has increased 10 times. Therefore for a 20 dB increase in sound intensity, although the sound intensity is 100 times greater, we perceive the sound as only 4 times as loud.[3]

How Bad Is My Hearing?

Hearing health care professionals classify hearing into several categories such as normal, slight, mild, moderate, moderately severe, severe, profound and deaf. Not all of them use all of these categories, nor do they all use the same hearing loss ranges in each one. In the past, most used this simple scale (Fig. 2-1).

Traditional Hearing Classification	
Hearing Classification Threshold	Hearing
Normal hearing	up to 20 dB
Mild hearing loss	20 to 40 dB
Moderate hearing loss	40 to 60 dB
Severe hearing loss	60 to 90 dB
Profound hearing loss	>90 dB

Fig. 2-1. The simple classification of hearing loss used in the past by many hearing health care professionals.

Today, research has shown that even hearing losses of only a few decibels can cause significant hearing problems. As a result, many hearing health care professionals have fine-tuned this scale to better reflect this reality (Fig. 2-2). (Note that these ranges are arbitrary and may vary slightly among authorities.)

Current Hearing Classification	
Hearing Classification Threshold	Hearing
Normal hearing	-10 to 15 dB
Slight hearing loss	16 to 25 dB
Mild hearing loss	26 to 40 dB
Moderate hearing loss	41 to 55 dB
Moderately severe hearing loss	56 to 70 dB
Severe hearing loss	71 to 90 dB
Profound hearing loss	91 to 120 dB
Deaf	above 120 dB[4,5]

Fig 2-2. The system of hearing loss classification used by many hearing health care professionals today.

If your audiologist tests your hearing and tells you that you have a bilateral (in both ears) hearing loss of 45 dB, you have a moderate hearing loss. If you have a 20 dB hearing loss, you would have a slight or mild hearing loss, depending on which classification system you use.

Don't let the terms "slight hearing loss" or "mild hearing loss" mislead you. You may think this means you don't have much of a hearing problem. Audiologists now recognise the negative effects of even slight hearing losses, particularly in children. Actually, a mild hearing loss can be quite significant in how you interact with others.

The following sections describe what you would hear and understand if your hearing loss fell in these various classes. Please understand that these examples apply specifically to those with high frequency sensorineural hearing losses (sometimes referred to as "ski slope" losses)—by far the most common kind of hearing loss (about 90 percent of those with hearing losses). However they still generally apply to the few of us with low-frequency hearing losses (reverse slope losses) and to those with conductive losses. And again, remember that all our hearing losses are unique. No one hears exactly like anyone else so it is hard to pigeon-hole someone exactly.

1.   **Slight hearing loss (16-25 dB)**. You may have difficulty hearing faint speech or distant speech. At 15 dB you can miss up to 10 percent of speech if the speaker is distant or if there is much background noise. Normally this only causes problems under very poor listening conditions. However, children in school could benefit from sound field amplification if their classroom is noisy or if sounds reverberate. They should sit close to the teacher.

2.   **Mild hearing loss (26-40 dB)**. You will normally hear quite well under ideal listening situations such as listening to one or two people in a quiet room. However, you will have difficulty hearing faint or distant speech. Even a 30 dB loss can cause you to miss 25 percent to 40 percent of speech. You will have difficulty hearing and understanding soft-spoken people (especially women and children). To you, conversation seems soft and muffled. People often seem to mumble when they talk.

The degree of hearing difficulty you experience depends on the amount of background noise, the distance you are from the speaker and your type of hearing loss. If your hearing loss is between 35 and 40 dB, without amplification you really have a profound communications barrier. You will miss 50 to 60 percent of group discussions, especially when

Hearing Loss Definitions

deaf, spelled with a lower case "d" is the physical condition—the inability to hear. It is the medical or audiological term applied to people with essentially no useful hearing. They are medically, but not culturally deaf. It also describes those who became deaf later in life but who do not identify with the Deaf culture. This term includes oral deaf and late deafened people.

Deaf, spelled with a capital "D" denotes a member of the Deaf culture. It is a sociological term that refers to people, whether deaf, hard of hearing, or hearing who willingly identify with and participate in the language, society and culture of Deaf people. The Deaf culture uses sign language when communicating with friends and at cultural events. They normally neither speechread nor speak. Often members of the Deaf culture were born deaf, became deaf very early in life or were hearing children born to Deaf parents.

Deafened or Late Deafened refers to people, whether originally hearing or hard of hearing, who lost their hearing (either gradually or suddenly) as adults. They communicate using speech and "hear" by speechreading supplemented with writing and sometimes by signing.

voices are faint or the speaker is not in your line of vision. You will miss many consonants. You may have trouble hearing people talking to you if they are more than 10 feet away. If there is any background noise, you will hear people talking but you won't be able to understand what they are saying. You will benefit from wearing hearing aids or using a personal FM system or sound field FM system in groups and classrooms. You need to sit close to the speaker and the speaker must have adequate light on his face so you can speechread him.

Hard of Hearing refers to people who have a hearing loss whether slight, mild, moderate, severe or profound. Hard of hearing people use speech to communicate and hear using their remaining hearing, supplemented with hearing aids, assistive listening devices and speechreading. If your hearing loss occurred later in life, it is sometimes referred to as "adventitious" or "acquired" hearing loss.

Hearing Impaired has a derogatory connotation and is no longer an acceptable term to many hard of hearing people. In its place use either the words "deaf" or "hard of hearing" depending on the degree of hearing loss.[6]

Oral Deaf refers to people who were either born deaf or became deaf very early in life, but whose primary method of communication is speech. These people are often excellent speech-readers for this is their main method of "hearing".

3.   **Moderate hearing loss (41-55 dB)**. Conversations sound very soft to you or are barely heard. Therefore, you constantly strain to hear. This means you have trouble hearing and understanding normal conversations even under ideal listening situations. You can hear reasonably well in face to face conversations at distances of 3 to 5 feet. Without amplification, the amount of speech you miss can be 50 percent to 75 percent if you have a 40 dB loss and 80 percent to 100 percent if your hearing loss is 50 dB. You have considerable difficulty hearing in noisy places. You often ask people to repeat what they just said. You may find that you hear people better when you can see their faces because you are beginning to speechread them. You turn up the radio or T.V. louder than normal. People may accuse you of not paying attention. Because you have to strain to hear, you

31

have trouble paying attention for long periods. Since you don't hear as many background sounds, you may begin to feel detached from your environment. You should wear hearing aids all the time. People may begin to notice that you have imperfect speech and an unusual quality in your voice. Speechreading and speech therapy are usually needed, especially in children.

4. **Moderately severe hearing loss (56-70 dB)**. You can't hear normal conversations. You communicate with great difficulty under all conditions. Without amplification, conversation must be very loud to understand. A 55 dB loss can cause you to miss up to 100 percent of speech. You find that both the background and foreground sounds blend into each other. You only hear when the speaker is within 3 to 5 feet, or is talking loudly. Conversations, even while wearing hearing aids, are limited to one person or to a small group. Nevertheless, you have marked difficulty hearing in groups. As a result, you feel detached from those around you. To others, you don't appear to be paying attention. People have to repeat a lot of what they say because you don't get it the first time. You need to wear hearing aids all the time. You also need to learn speechreading and other coping strategies. You will likely have reduced speech intelligibility and voice quality unless you work with a speech therapist.

5. **Severe hearing loss (71-90 dB)**. You wear your hearing aids but you still miss a lot of conversations. With optimal amplification you hear loud environmental noises and detect the sounds of speech. However, you find it difficult to understand what was said. You find that speechreading is vital in order to understand everyday speech. If you can't see the speaker's face, you miss much of what he says. You hear loud speech about 1 foot from your

ear. Even then, what you hear may be distorted. You likely hear most vowel sounds but just as likely don't hear the consonants anymore. You often ignore people speaking around you because you can't understand them. Instead, you like to talk one to one in a quiet place. You often avoid social activities because you are ignored since you can't understand much of what is said. Your speech will likely deteriorate in quality, and in time become atonal or flat unless you work with a speech therapist in order to prevent this.

6.   **Profound hearing loss (91-120 dB)**. You are now considered "deaf." You may hear some loud sounds. Actually, you will be more aware of vibrations than tonal patterns. You wear hearing aids so you can hear your own voice. They also alert you to loud environmental noises. However, you have great difficulty hearing conversations even with your hearing aids. You do not rely on your hearing as the primary means of communication. You may use a combination of hearing aids, speechreading, writing on a notepad and American Sign Language to converse with others. You use your eyes more than your ears when communicating. For you, training in speechreading, speech therapy, and counselling is absolutely essential. Your speech will likely be of poor quality unless you continually practice speech therapy. You may be a good candidate for a cochlear implant.[7,8,9,10,11]

Hearing Loss Is Not Measured in Percentage!

Hearing loss is not measured as a percentage. We measure it in decibels (dB). The reason you want to be aware of this is because so often people talk about

How This Percentage Business Happened

Where did the idea come from that we can measure hearing loss in percentages? Here is how Brad Ingrao, an audiologist who really understands these things, explained it.

"To measure Sound Pressure Level (SPL) you need to do a logarithmic calculation that is so strange that 20 + 20 = 26 (dB SPL).

To make a scale that makes sense to most people (including us knucklehead audiologists), a different equation is used to convert the SPL scale to the Hearing Level (HL) scale that goes from 0 dB HL (normal threshold) to 120 dB HL (pain).

If we forget about the 120 (most people tend to avoid that), we get 0 dB to 100 dB as a usable (dynamic) range of hearing for the average 'normal' ear.

Since doctors and audiologists tend to under-estimate their patient's ability to understand such things (or they don't understand it themselves), the erroneous concept of dB = % evolved."

This is just plain nonsense. The problem is that a 50 dB loss means you'll miss over 90 percent of average speech—not just 50 percent as you might expect.

having a 50 percent hearing loss when in fact they have a 50 dB loss. For some reason, we often equate dB units with percentage points. This is absolutely wrong because the dB scale, like the Richter (Moment Magnitude) scale used for measuring earthquake intensities, is open-ended. Because there is no end, you can't calculate a percentage.

However, even if you assumed that 100 dB equalled 100 percent, 50 percent would not equal

50 dB—not by a long shot. 50 percent would be, believe it or not, 97 dB! Likewise, 50 dB, when compared to 100 dB, is not just half as loud, but would only be one thousandth of one percent as loud! Now you can see why you must get out of the habit of using percentages when talking about your hearing loss. They are absolutely meaningless!

For example, I have a 80 dB loss. Therefore, the softest sound I can hear in the voice range needs to be 100,000,000 times louder than the softest sound you can hear if your hearing is normal. (Note that 1 in 100,000,000 is definitely not 80 per cent!) That gives you an idea of just how bad my hearing is.

I know that we like to use laymen's terms, so why not just say that you have a severe hearing loss or whatever. It is much more meaningful, not to mention, far more accurate.

Mumble, Mutter, Muddle—Here's Why We Hear the Way We Do

People with normal hearing often wonder why we cannot understand them if we can hear them talking. "Just turn up your hearing aids," they unwittingly say. They don't realize that volume alone is not the answer.

In order to understand speech we need two different abilities. First, we need the ability to detect (hear) speech sounds. If we don't hear a sound, it doesn't have any meaning for us. Second, we need the ability to interpret what we have heard. We have difficulty understanding speech when we no longer hear all the sounds of speech—typically the softer sounds. When this happens many words sound alike to us. We may have trouble interpreting the word "thin." We might have thought you said "chin," "fin," "kin," "pin," "sin," "shin" or "tin." In this case, we don't need more volume, we need more clarity.

We will look at hearing loss first. As an audiologist tests your hearing, she plots your results on an audiogram (Fig. 2-3). An audiogram is just a graph or

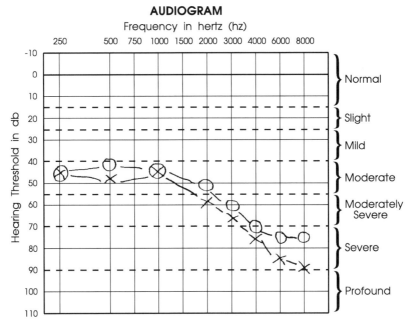

Fig. 2-3. This is an audiogram of a person with a moderate hearing loss in the lower frequencies. This hearing loss increases to a severe loss at the high frequencies. This person's right (O) ear hears marginally better than the left (X) ear.

picture of your hearing loss. Here is how you read it. Along the left side, it shows hearing threshold levels. This shows how loud a sound has to be before you can just hear it. Across the top is the frequency of the sounds you are tested for. The testing range is between 250 Hz (although you may be able to hear down to about 18 Hz) and 8,000 Hz (although normal ears can hear up to about 20,000 Hz or even higher).

Audiologists test you in this particular range because speech and normal environmental sounds are in this range of frequencies. (I have added the different hearing loss classifications along the right side of the audiogram—and the dashed lines—so you can understand it better.)

What Your Pets Hear

Have you ever wondered what frequencies of sound your pets hear? In contrast to the upper human limit of 18,000 to 20,000 Hz, cats hear sounds up to 25,000 Hz and man's best friend, your pooch, can hear sounds as high as 35,000 Hz.[12] Now you know.

As your audiologist tests your hearing, he marks your hearing thresholds for each frequency tested. He uses a blue "X" for your left ear and a red "O" for your right ear. He then joins the X's and O's with short lines. If the "X" is in the "O", both of your ears have the same hearing threshold for that frequency of sound.

Fig. 2-3 shows the results of a person with a moderate hearing loss at the lower frequencies. This person's hearing then dramatically drops down to

Different Losses at Different Pitches

Classifying hearing losses as mild, moderate, severe, etc. is convenient but does not tell the whole story. Normally, we have different amounts of hearing at different frequencies. For example, you may have a severe loss for high frequency sounds, but only a mild loss at the lower frequencies. Or you generally may have normal hearing with a moderate loss at only one frequency, typical of the "notch" produced by noise-induced hearing loss.

a severe loss at the higher frequencies. Up to 1,000 Hz, the curve is relatively flat (a "flat" curve) and then drops off and becomes a "ski slope" curve indicating a precipitous hearing loss.

Now lets look at what happens to your hearing as you get older. Typically, as you age your hearing first begins to drop off at the higher frequencies, then the mid-frequencies and finally (and to a much lesser extent) the low frequencies. The medical term for this is presbycusis (press-be-COO-sis). If your hearing loss is a combination of both ageing and noise, doctors may use the term sociocusis[13] (so-see-oh-COO-sis). Sociocusis is probably far more common than presbycusis since we are all exposed to loud noises

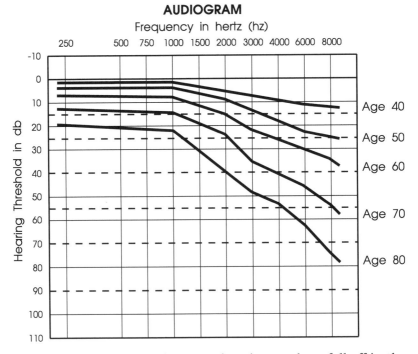

Fig. 2-4. As you grow older, your hearing tends to fall off in the higher frequencies. Doctors call this presbycusis. Your hearing loss normally gets progressively worse as you age.

from time to time although the more common term is presbycusis. Fig. 2-4 shows how your hearing loss may look at various ages.[14] Note that these curves are averages. Your specific curve may look much different. Some people hardly have any hearing loss, even into old age. Other people's ears age far more rapidly than these curves might suggest.

Fig. 2-5 shows the "speech banana" superimposed on a blank audiogram. The "speech banana" is the area of an audiogram that the various speech sounds cover. (We call it this because it looks much like the silhouette of a banana.) Inside this "speech banana" I have located the various speech sounds (letters).[15,16] Their positions on the audiogram shows both their relative

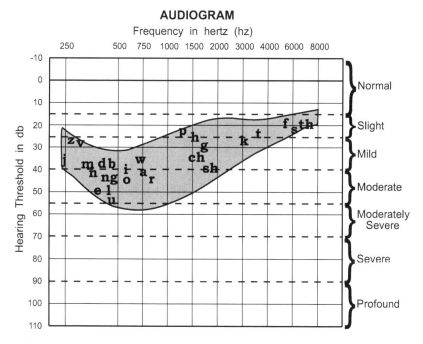

Fig. 2-5. The "speech banana" shows the frequency and volume of each speech sound (letter). The vowels are louder and clustered near the 500 Hz line. The consonants tend to be softer and higher in frequency.

loudness and their frequency. We will see why this is so important in a minute.

Notice that the vowels (a, e, i, o, u) cluster near 500 Hz while many of the consonants (the rest of the letters in the alphabet) range up to 8,000 Hz. Also note that the vowels tend to be louder. They have a hearing threshold of between 40 and 55 dB. The consonants are softer and generally range between about 20 and 40 dB. In order to hear speech properly we must be able to hear the softest sounds **and** the loudest sounds as well.

Because vowels are strong, low-frequency sounds, you can hear them at a distance. They also penetrate background noise. The weaker, higher-pitched consonants, on the other hand, fade out quickly as the distance increases and get lost in any background noise.

Women Hear Better Than Men

Did you know that above 1,000 Hz, women hear better than men? Their high frequency losses are not as great as in men at all age levels.

For example, by age 60, women have an average loss of 25 dB at 4,000 Hz. Men, on the other hand, have a 55 dB loss at the same age and frequency.[17]

As you get older, you lose your high frequencies faster than your low frequencies (Fig. 2-4). This means that although you still hear the vowels, you no longer hear many of the consonants (because they are higher in frequency and are softer in volume). Therefore, if you have a 40 dB loss, (much like the person in Fig. 2-3) you typically will not hear the consonants (20–40 dB). You will mainly just hear the vowels (40–55 dB).

AUDIOGRAM

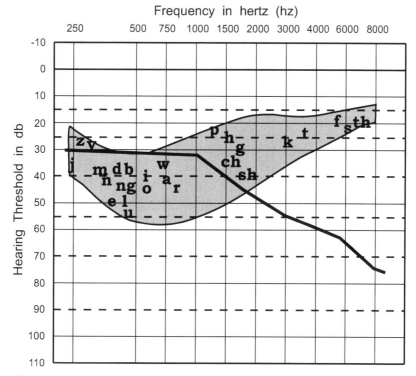

Fig. 2-6. This audiogram shows a person with a mild hearing loss at the lower frequencies. His hearing loss becomes worse at the higher frequencies. He can no longer hear speech sounds (letters) above the line. This distorts the way speech sounds and makes understanding speech difficult.

The audiogram in Fig. 2-6 shows the hearing loss of a person with a mild (30 dB) hearing loss at the low frequencies. This loss drops off more and more towards the higher frequencies. The sounds of any letters above the line would be too faint to hear. For this person, only the sounds of the letters below this line would be loud enough for him to hear clearly. Because so many speech sounds are too soft to hear, anything you say to this person will sound distorted. Very likely he won't understand much of what you say.

Fig. 2-7 shows those parts of three sentences (each line is a sentence) that a person with such a hearing loss typically might hear. Look at these sentences. Imagine that someone comes up to you and utters these sounds. What would you think he

I	u	own	ree
W	a	im i	i
Don	a	a	an

Fig. 2-7. This is what you would hear if you had the mild hearing loss with presbycusis shown in Fig. 2-6. You would hear people talking but would not be able to understand much of what they are saying. (See Fig. 2-8 on page 44 for what he really said.)

had said to you? This is the gibberish hard of hearing people hear all the time. Shocking, isn't it?

Here is another way of understanding why hard of hearing people have difficulty comprehending what you say. Let's look at some interesting but relatively unknown facts that relate to understanding speech.

In the English alphabet, there are 5 vowels and 21 consonants. The vowels comprise about 20 percent of the alphabet. This means the 21 consonants obviously comprise the remaining 80 percent of the alphabet.

Now, what percent of all the energy you use in talking do you think the vowels use? If you guessed 20 percent you made the obvious, logical decision. However, you would be totally wrong! Here is the shocking truth. Those five vowels actually consume a whopping 95 percent of your speech energy. This means that the 21 consonants together only use a minuscule 5 percent of your speech energy.

Breaking this down further, 60 percent of speech energy occurs below 500 Hz. Usually, these are the vowel sounds. The medium frequency sounds, between

500 and 1,000 Hz, contribute about 35 percent of the speech energy. The higher frequency speech components, which are so critical to understanding speech have very little energy, only a minuscule 5 percent (Fig. 2-9).

Now follow this. In terms of intelligibility, sounds lower than 500 Hz only contribute 5 percent to overall speech intelligibility. Sounds between 500 and 1,000

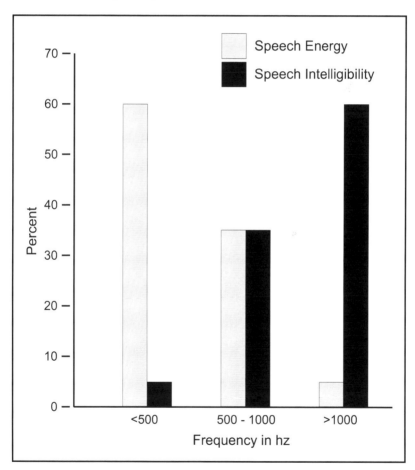

Fig. 2-9. Speech energy is mostly in the lower frequencies (grey bars) while speech intelligibility is mostly in the higher frequencies (black bars). As a result, hearing loss affects the intelligibility of speech far more than it would appear it should when only looking at the actual hearing loss.

Hz contribute 35 percent to speech intelligibility, whereas sounds above 1,000 Hz contribute a whopping 60 percent to speech intelligibility (Fig. 2-9).[18]

| Is the phone free? |
| What time is it? |
| Don't take a chance. |

Fig. 2-8. What was really said in Fig. 2-7.

We all need to hear those vitally important high-frequency consonant sounds in order to understand speech. Also, remember, those of us with sensorineural hearing losses have damaged hair cells in our cochleae. Unfortunately, it is the hair cells for the consonant frequencies that suffer the most damage. Now follow this. As we have seen, English has four times more consonants than vowels. Also, each consonant is composed of several frequencies. Therefore, there is about a one in five chance that these "bad" hair cells will also affect about one in five consonantal frequencies. This means that we also have a one in five chance of misunderstanding any given phrase. The conversations we hear are filled with

Only Vowels Really Raise the Volume

Whether you yell or whisper, the higher frequency consonants remain at much the same volume. The lower frequency consonants increase a little in volume. It is just the vowels that get really loud.

Go ahead. Try it. First whisper the word "stop." Notice how loud the letters "s," "t" and "p" sound. Now call out loudly "stop." Notice that those three letters are still at the same loudness level as they were when you whispered. However, the vowel sound "o" is another matter. It is far louder when you yell. Interesting, isn't it?[19]

hundreds of tiny gaps. This causes distorted speech. In short, for us, language often falls apart.[20]

Without consonants, our language would just sound like a lot of gibberish. We'd all sound like we were talking with our mouths full of marbles.

You don't have to be a rocket scientist to realize that as you lose your hearing, you will only hear the louder sounds. So which sounds will you hear? The vowels of course.

Look at Fig. 2-10. It contains three sentences (one per line) showing only the loud vowel sounds you, as a hard of hearing person, normally hear. Can you decipher them? Do you even have the faintest clue as to what that person is saying? All that comes out sounds much like someone chanting.

o	a	ui	e a	o i			
u	a	a	a	o a	i	u	
u	oo a	a e	u	e	u	a	

Fig. 2-10. If all you can hear are the vowels, there is no way you can understand what a speaker is saying, is there?

Although the vowels are what we, as hard of hearing people, typically hear, by themselves they don't contribute all that much to the intelligibility of speech. We can hear you talking, but don't have a clue as to what you are saying!

With just the consonants, it's another story. You probably can quickly figure out the exact meaning of the sentence with only the consonants. Fig. 2-11 gives the same three sentences that baffled you in

Fig. 2-10. Go ahead. See how easy it is to figure them out. (You can check your results in Fig. 2-12 at the bottom of this page.)

C m   s q ckly s p ss bl .

Th   m n r n f st t c tch h s b s.

Th   f tb ll pl y r f mbl d th   b ll.

Fig. 2-11. If you could only hear the consonants, a little effort would allow you to figure out what was said. This shows that most of speech intelligibility is contained in the consonants which hard of hearing people don't hear well, if they hear them at all.

Now you understand a little better why we have trouble understanding you even though we hear you talking. We hear the vowels and a few of the consonants. Yet, in order to understand speech, we desperately need to hear those soft-spoken consonants as well. If we can't hear them, we just hear so much gibber-jabber.

I'll bet you are thinking, "If a hard of hearing person hears the low frequency sounds but can't hear the high frequency sounds, there is a simple solution." Obviously, all someone needs to do is invent a new hearing aid that would amplify high frequency sounds while leaving low frequency sounds alone. Then we could hear normally.

Come as quickly as possible.

The man ran fast to catch his bus.

The football player fumbled the ball.

Fig. 2-12. What was really said in Fig. 2-10 and the complete message of Fig. 2-11.

Good thinking! Surprise! That is exactly what most modern hearing aids do. But do the people using them hear normally? No, we do not. We may hear better, but not normally. This is because there are other insidious factors at work in our ears.

It's Hard To Hear If You Are Hard of Hearing

As you begin to lose your hearing, something happens that you probably didn't expect. Hearing (or more correctly, understanding what you are hearing) becomes more and more difficult. Being hard of hearing is hard! Volume alone is not the problem. Even with hearing aids, it is still difficult, and sometimes impossible, to understand speech in certain situations. Here is why.

Here's Why Our Hearing Gets "Fuzzy"

We have been taught that our auditory nerves only carry messages from our inner ears to our brains. This is not true. Our brains also send messages to our inner ears from at least three different parts—our thinking part, our emotional part and our reflex-action part. These signals fine-tune our inner ears.

Aging and noise affects these fine-tuning nerves as much as it does our hearing nerves. When our inner ears are no longer fine-tuned, the sounds reaching our brains get distorted. They sound "fuzzy." That is partially why we no longer understand what we are hearing.[21]

If we have inner ear (sensorineural) hearing losses, we have not just one, but at least four factors working against us. First, because some (or many) of the hair cells in our inner ears have died, our ears lose their sensitivity to sound. This means we need more volume. Second, the lack of these same hair cells causes our ears to lose their ability to accurately separate or discriminate between these different sounds. Third, we don't hear sounds at their correct relative volumes. Some sounds are now too soft to hear and others are much too loud! (See the section on "Recruitment" for a fuller explanation of points 2 and 3.) Fourth, our auditory nerves lose some of their "fine-tuning" ability. (See text box on previous page.) Combined, these four factors make understanding speech most difficult.

Discrimination

Those of us with sensorineural hearing losses (this applies to about 90 percent of adults with hearing losses) lose, to some degree, our ability to distinguish one sound from another. The proper term for this is "discrimination." Discrimination allows us to understand speech. Without it, speech sounds fuzzy and all mushed together. As we get older, this inordinate reduction in discrimination causes us so much trouble understanding speech.

In case you're wondering, audiologists determine how well we discriminate between sounds (distinguish one sound from another) by determining the percentage of phonetically-balanced single-syllable words from a special list we correctly recognize when they are spoken at a comfortable loudness.

Ninety percent and higher is considered normal. If your discrimination score is between 75 percent and 90 percent, you will have mild difficulty understanding speech, especially if there is any background noise. However, your brain will normally still be able to fill in the gaps and figure out what was said. If your discrimination score drops to between 60 percent and

75 percent, you will experience moderate difficulty understanding speech. Your will find conversations difficult to follow because speech often seems distorted. If you can only discriminate between 45 percent and 60 percent of the words you hear, you will have a tough time understanding speech unless you supplement what you hear with speechreading. If you score below 45 percent you will find that speech sounds more like a foreign language than anything else. You will have severe difficulty understanding much of anything.

Percentages vs. Decibels

Hearing and understanding what you hear are two different things.

Hearing loss is measured in decibels, not as a percentage. Therefore, you can say you have a 70 dB hearing loss, but not a 70 percent loss.

Discrimination ability, however, is measured as a percentage. So if you have a discrimination score of 70 percent, you understand 70 out of every 100 words spoken to you (at a volume you can comfortably hear.)

So, remember, how much you **hear** is measured in decibels. How much you **understand** of what you hear is measured as a percentage.

We have two separate problems with discrimination. First, as we saw previously, we usually don't hear the high-frequency sounds such as **ch**, **f**, **k**, **p**, **s**, **sh**, **t** and **th** distinctly. As a result we have a lot of blanks it try and fill in. At the same time, because of our damaged inner ears, what we do hear sounds fuzzy. We are never certain what we hear. For example, the words "cop," "hop," "pot," "sought," "shop" or "thought" all sound about the same to us. This means that we hear you talking but cannot always understand what you say. Many times what we hear doesn't make sense. To us it is mostly a bunch of gibber-jabber. Simply repeating these words seldom helps if volume alone is not the problem. We still hear garbled sounds. So be patient when we misunderstand you (Fig. 2-13). Our ears no longer give us the correct message.

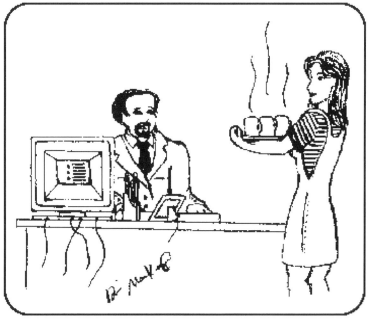

Fig. 2-13. "Thank you Jane, but I said 5 copies, not 5 coffees."

To show you just how easy it is for us to misunderstand you, at college one day, my daughter, Jennifer, who is hard of hearing (wonder where she got it from?) was talking with a friend in a parking lot in the pouring rain. He actually had asked her if she would ever **cheat** on her boyfriend. She smiled and replied, "Yes, all the time!" By the startled look on his face she knew that something wasn't quite right. What she had understood him to say was, "Would you ever do something **sweet** for your boyfriend!"

On top of discrimination problems, people with sensorineural hearing losses may also have problems with pitch distortion. Certain tones may sound higher or lower to us than they really are. Then, too, one of our ears may hear the tones normally, while the other one hears the same tones higher or lower or perceives them as noises instead of pure tones.[22] This makes understanding speech even more difficult. But this is not all, we also have problems with recruitment!

What Did You Say?

"I know you believe you understand what you think I said, but I'm not sure you realise that what you thought you heard is not what I said."

That's us all right!

Recruitment

All those of us with sensorineural hearing losses face another daunting headache—sounds get too loud too fast. Yes, you heard it right. Even though we have hearing losses, some sounds that people with normal hearing find comfortable become painfully loud to us. The technical name for this predictable distortion in our perception of loudness goes by the name of "recruitment."[23] As a general rule, the more severe our hearing loss, the greater this abnormal loudness growth becomes.

Recruitment may seem to be a funny name for this phenomenon. Probably you think of recruitment when the government runs short of military personnel and puts on a recruitment drive. If it becomes necessary, your brain does this too. When the hair cells in your cochlea are damaged or die, your brain takes action to replace their functions. Simply put, it recruits the hair cells on each side of the dead ones to help do the job. Thus the name recruitment.

Here is how it works. Each hair cell in our ears vibrates at a different frequency. Rather than working independently, these hair cells work together in groups called critical bands. Each critical band is about 16 percent wider than its central frequency. (For example, a tone of 1,000 Hz. [cycles] would have a critical band of 160 Hz. surrounding it.) We perceive the frequency of a given sound depending on which critical bands are stimulated. How loud we hear a given sound depends on how many critical bands that sound stimulates.[24]

When something happens to damage or kill some of our hair cells (such as old age, loud noise, or certain medications) we lose a corresponding amount of our hearing. As more of our hair cells die, we progressively lose more of our hearing. So guess what? Our brains automatically widen the critical bands to try to make up for these lost hair cells. They recruit the living hair cells on each side of the dead ones. As a result, some critical bands now overlap. This means that instead of just one critical band being stimulated for a given sound, now two or more may be stimulated. This creates at least three further problems for us.

In the following example, let's assume that three critical bands are now stimulated when only one would have been stimulated if hearing had been normal. What happens? First, it affects our discrimination because we can no longer distinguish between closely related frequencies of sounds. This affects our ability to hear the difference between similar-sounding words. Consequently, many words now sound alike.

We may hear you talking but can't tell exactly what words you are saying.

Second, the volume of a given sound is no longer normal. This is because the number of critical bands stimulated by a given sound largely determines how loud we hear that sound. For example a sound that stimulates two critical bands is twice as loud as a sound that only stimulates one. So, in our example where three critical bands are stimulated instead of one, a person with a hearing loss would hear this sound three times louder than normal. This makes listening to these sounds very uncomfortable.

Third, because of our hearing losses and these shifts in our critical bands, sounds appear to us to increase far more rapidly than they do in people with normal hearing. A small change in sound intensity produces a very big change in our ears since more nerve fibres are switched on or recruited. This is related to our reduced dynamic range.

Your dynamic range is that area between the softest sound you can hear and the loudest sound you can stand. For example, a person with normal hearing can hear extremely quiet sounds between 0 and 20 dB. At the top end of the scale, they can tolerate very loud sounds without discomfort up to about 115 dB. Thus, the dynamic range for people with normal hearing is about 95 dB (115 - 20 = 95). The dynamic range of people with a sensorineural hearing loss is typically much narrower than the range for those with normal hearing (Fig. 2-14).

A person with a 75 dB hearing loss only has a dynamic range of about 30 dB. This is because he cannot hear the soft sounds you can. At the same time, he cannot tolerate sounds as loud as you can.

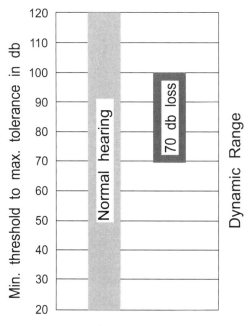

Fig. 2-14. The dynamic range of a hard of hearing person is much less than that of a normally-hearing person. The worse the hearing loss, the smaller the dynamic range.

This means that all the sounds he hears are compressed into a narrow band. As a result, some sounds are uncomfortably loud to him while people with normal hearing are not bothered by these same sounds. Also, dropping your voice slightly (as you perceive it) will drop it right through the bottom of his dynamic range, and he will hear nothing.

The loudness of sounds increases much faster for us than for people with normal hearing. For example, if you have normal hearing, and you hear a sound at 55 dB (normal conversation volume) and then hear this same sound at 65 dB, you will perceive the second sound as being about twice as loud as the first sound. However, if you have a hearing loss of 75 dB, this actual increase of 10 dB doesn't just sound twice as loud. It sounds about 7 or 8 times as loud (Fig. 2-15)! This is what recruitment can be like. What seems just a bit louder to you may be painfully loud to us.

Recruitment is also one reason why we miss the punch line of jokes so often. When people come to the punch line of jokes, they typically lower their voices for emphasis. Let's assume they drop the volume at

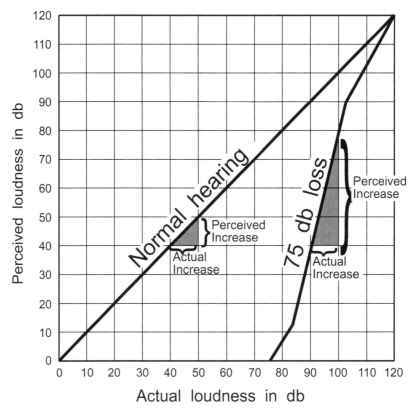

Fig. 2-15. The greater the hearing loss, the greater the perceived increase in sound for a given actual sound increase. In this case, the perceived sound level for the person with a hearing loss appears to be about 8 times louder while a person with normal hearing would perceive the same sound increase as only twice as loud.

which they were speaking in half—from 55 dB to 45 dB—which is still at a normal conversational volume. If you have normal hearing, you have no trouble hearing this—it just sounds about half as loud to you, but it is still well within your dynamic range. However, for someone like me, the person is not now talking half as loud, but only about one eighth as loud! It actually drops through the bottom of our dynamic range. Essentially, we don't even hear them talking any more!

The result is that we have heard most of the main part of the joke; are frustrated because we couldn't hear the punch line; and then are deafened by the terribly loud (to us) laughter that ensues.

Since recruitment has to do with the ramifications of hair cells dying, people with conductive hearing losses, such as otosclerosis, do not have to worry about recruitment. This is because conductive hearing losses occur in the middle ear, not the inner ear where the hair cells are.

If you have a sensorineural hearing loss however, you have problems with recruitment to some degree or other, whether you know it or not. In fact, all people with a sensorineural hearing loss exhibit this abnormally steep loudness growth. This is because the reduced dynamic range means the loudness function must be steeper than normal. Typically, your recruitment will be the worst at the frequency of your greatest hearing loss. A frequent misconception is that recruitment refers only to the less frequent cases of hypersensitivity to high intensity sounds.[25]

Some of us have recruitment problems to the extreme. A small increase in loudness sounds to us like you just went from a whisper to a shout. For a person with severe recruitment, one sound may be perfectly comfortable, while another, only slightly louder, may sound like a jet plane taking off directly overhead. This is a real phenomenon and not one to be laughed at or taken lightly. It can hurt! I know. This is why people with hearing loss may perceive slightly louder sounds as too loud. When you speak to them and they don't hear you, you raise you voice a bit, then they complain, "Don't shout at me, I'm not deaf!"[26]

For those of us with severe hearing losses, recruitment means that the perceived loudness increases much faster as sound levels increase. Because of this rapid build-up of the sensation of loudness, as soon as sounds become loud enough to be heard, just a little more increase in loudness brings pain. That is why certain levels of loudness hurt our ears, even though people with normal hearing are perfectly comfortable with the same sounds.[27] In extreme cases, by the time a sound is loud enough for us to hear, it is already almost too loud for us to stand. The dynamic range in this case is almost down to 0 dB.

Incidentally, people with severe recruitment almost always have tinnitus.

This abnormally rapid growth in loudness makes speech difficult to understand. A small change in speech loudness can make an enormous difference in how well we will understand what is said. To us, weak sounds drop into silence. At the same time, sounds that are loud to people with normal hearing are also loud to us.[28] This recruitment factor, plus our inability to hear consonant sounds, makes it particularly difficult for us to hear speech in noisy surroundings.[29]

We wear hearing aids to try to hear better. The overall aim of hearing aids is to restore normal loudness at all levels and frequencies, and thus make speech sound more natural.[30] However, it is hard to do this because the wide dynamic range of conversational speech does not fit into the restricted dynamic range of our hearing loss. Therefore, even with hearing aids with wide dynamic range compression, some parts of speech are still below our hearing threshold. This causes speech to sound blurred and "mumbley." However, if additional high-frequency amplification is added to counteract this tendency, loud sounds may become unpleasantly harsh.

Chapter 2 Endnotes

1   Vernick, 1993. p. 8.
2   Engel, 1993. pp. 159.
3   Olsson, 1996. p. 4.
4   Shimon, 1992. p. 27.
5   Staab, 1991. p. 30.
6   Warick, 1997. p.9.
7   Staab, 1991, pp. 30-31.
8   Alpiner, 1987. pp. 436-437.
9   Rezen, 1985. p. 23.
10 Shimon, 1992. p. 54.
11 Children and Youth with a Hearing Loss, 1994. pp. 169-170.
12 Vernick, 1993. p. 13.
13 Vernick, 1993. p. 38.
14 Shimon, 1992. p. 51.
15 Shimon, 1992. p. 52.
16 Alpiner, 1987. p. 310.
17 Staab, 1991. p. 43.
18 In The Ear Rationale, 1983. p. 6.
19 Olsson, 1996. p. 4.
20 Huning, 1992. p. 39.
21 Olsson, 1996. p. 3.
22 Helleberg, 1980. p. 41.
23 Ingrao, 1996. p. 1.
24 Ingrao, 1997. p. 1.
25 Pluvinage, 1992. p. 6.
26 Vernick, 1993. p. 38.
27 Helleberg, 1980. p. 104.
28 Waldhauer, 1988. p. 2.
29 Helleberg, 1980. p. 41.
30 Waldhauer, 1988. p. 2.

Chapter 3

The Wages of Din Is Deaf—Things You Should Know About Noise and Hearing Loss

Excessive Noise

The pervading noise in our industrialized society causes a staggering amount of hearing loss, especially among teens and adults. Rock concerts, boom boxes (and boom cars) and walk-around stereos (iPods, MP3 players, etc.) are endangering the hearing of an entire generation. One study recently revealed that nearly one third of students entering college already have a detectable hearing loss![1,2]

Another study reported that those students who had listened to an average of 2,000 hours of loud music had more damage than those who had only listened for about 225 hours in the same period did. The heavy listeners showed a 10 to 20 percent deterioration in their ability to hear certain sounds, especially when background noise was present.[3] A British study of young adults between 15 and 23 found that those who regularly used portable personal stereos **and** attended rock concerts had **double** the rate of hearing loss when compared to others their own age. Some of the little personal stereos can produce sounds as loud as 126 dB—that's equivalent to someone using a jackhammer in your ears![4]

Today, noise is the most common reason for hearing loss in people between the ages of 20 and 40. However, audiologists are now seeing more and more noise-induced hearing loss in young people between the ages of 10 and 20![5] Tragic isn't it? These young people now have to go through life with a hearing loss that never should have occurred.

However, try telling a teenager that they are damaging their hearing by listening to excessively loud music and you are immediately identified as out of touch. But just ask how many of them have left a school dance with their ears ringing, and nearly all of them will admit they have.[6] Our ears ring in response to excessive noise. They are trying to tell us they have been hurt. They are bruised although we can't see any black and blue marks on them.

A recent survey of 400 youths in France revealed that 1 out of every 5 of them suffers from hearing loss. A similar study a decade earlier showed that only 1 out of 10 young people suffered such a loss. Because of this, the French National Assembly voted to limit the sound level from personal stereos to 100 dB.

According to ear surgeon, Jean-Pierre Cave, volumes above 100 dB can result in permanent damage in just a few hours. It takes only minutes for such damage to occur when the volume is above

115 dB, and many personal stereos can easily produce these volumes.

Rock concerts may be hurting even more young people than personal stereos according to French hearing specialist, Christian Meyer-Bisch. Indeed, regular attendees of rock concerts had significant hearing loss compared with healthy 18-year-olds. No wonder French National Assembly deputy Jean-Francois Matter warned, "We're producing a generation of deaf people".[7]

It's not just young people who wear personal stereos. Many adults wear them to block out background noise. For example, they wear them in noisy factories. The result is that their ears not only have to contend with the background noise, but also the additional sounds of the music they are listening to. Together these boost the sounds in their ears to dangerous levels. Therefore, never use headphones to try to drown out other noise. Be smart and use proper ear protectors or get away from the racket.

Noise is a leading occupational hazard. Some of the noisiest jobs are found in the primary industries such as mining, logging, farming, and drilling, as well as in mills, manufacturing plants and construction sites. People who work in these trades or around noisy equipment are at risk of losing their hearing.

Remember, excessive noise is the most common cause of hearing loss in adults under 50.[8] The tragedy is that a lot of this hearing loss could be prevented. We just need to protect our ears when we can't get away from this racket. Excessively loud sounds are all around us. Appliances in the home, loud music, lawn mowers, snowmobiles, power tools and sporting

Approximately How Loud Sounds Are

Sound level	Activity causing sound	Loudness rating
180 dB	Roar of rocket blasting off	Instant permanent
140 dB	Shotgun/rifle blast	hearing loss
	Jet 100 feet away at take-off	
130 dB	Firecrackers	Threshold of pain
120 dB	Jackhammer, pneumatic drill	
	Severe thunder	
	Hockey crowd	
	Siren	
110 dB	Car horn	
	Amplified rock music	
	Chain saw	Uncomfortably loud
100 dB	Snowmobile	
	Farm tractor	
	Subway train, Elevated train	
	Blender	
	Power lawn mower	
90 dB	Shop tools	
	Heavy city traffic	
	Person shouting from 2 feet away	
	Diesel truck 40 mph 50 feet away	
	Noisy factory	Loud
80 dB	Garbage disposal	
	Crowded restaurant	
	Alarm clock	
	Water running in sink	
	Average factory	
	Vacuum cleaner	
	City traffic	
	Loud voice	Moderately loud
70 dB	Passenger car 50 mph 50 feet away	
60 dB	Singing birds	
	Window air conditioner	
	Quiet automobile	
	Typewriter	
	Sewing machine	
50 dB	Average office	
	Normal conversation	Quiet
40 dB	Refrigerator	
	Quiet office	Very quiet

30 dB	Average home	
	Quiet library	
	Dripping tap	
	Whisper 5 feet away	
20 dB	Light rainfall	
	Rustle of leaves	
10 dB	Very faint whisper	Just audible
0 dB	Softest sound human ears can hear	

weapons all take their daily toll. Listening to any of these loud sounds for long periods eventually causes permanent sensorineural hearing loss.

Excessive noise damages our ears in one of two ways. Intense sound waves—like from a nearby explosion—can actually blast away the vital hair cells in our inner ears and leave us instantly and permanently with a hearing loss.

Also, intense sounds can provoke a stress reaction in our bodies. When this happens our blood pressure rises in our body core while blood circulation to our extremities including our ears decreases. If the noise (and stress reaction) continues for more than a few minutes, our ears are deprived of the oxygen they need. This makes our hair cells even more sensitive to noise damage.[9]

Incidentally, for some reason men are more susceptible to hearing loss from loud noises than women. They sustain greater hearing loss than women working along side of them in the same noisy environments do.[10]

Hear Today, Gone Tomorrow—Safe Sound Levels

Perhaps you are now curious. You want to know exactly how much noise your ears can safely stand. Most governments have established minimum noise standards that industries must follow. (See text box.)

Permissible Sound Levels (Old)

Here are the older permissible noise level standards that governments used to think your ears could stand without permanent damage.[11] Notice that the sound level increases are all in 5 dB steps.

Sound level dB(A)	Hours /day
85	8
90	4
95	2
100	1
105	30 min
110	15 min.
115	8 min.

First, note that these are the minimum standards. Why try to go as close to that line as possible? It's your hearing that is at risk, not someone else's. Second, the permissible exposure for given noise levels gets revised downwards from time to time. This means that noise levels that once were acceptable have now been found to cause hearing loss. That's another good reason to stay away from the minimum standards. For example, some researchers feel that even our current standards are too liberal. They suggest that even 5 minutes at 110 dB will lead to some hearing loss.[12]

The currently suggested level where hearing protection should begin is 85 dB. (Your power lawn-mower runs at about 90 dB. So does the blender in your kitchen.) According to hearing experts, ear protection should be mandatory at 90 dB. It's ironic, isn't it, that governments try to enforce the use of ear protection for industrial work at 85 dB while at the same time condoning much higher noise levels for pleasure from discos, rock bands and personal stereos.[13] We are talking about noise levels of 100 dB, 110 dB and even more. (A jackhammer operates around 120 dB. Such noise levels will cause hearing damage within minutes.)

Permissible Sound Levels (Current)

Governments are now mostly using stricter standards that use 3 dB steps, which more accurately reflects how sound levels and time interact with our ears. When you increase the sound level by 3 dB, you halve the safe time you can be exposed to this noise.

Sound level dB(A)	Hours /day
85	8
88	4
91	2
94	1
97	30 min.
100	15 min.
103	8 min.

Let's get sensible and refuse to put up with this nonsense. I have measured sound levels of up to 115 dB in business rallies where they played loud music for up to an hour before the meetings began, and from time to time throughout the meetings. This is ridiculous. These are sound levels up to 1,000 times louder than those known to cause hearing loss. Remember, I'm talking about a business rally, not a rock concert! I repeatedly asked them to tone it down. When they refused, I soon left that organization. What real gain is there in making money, but losing my hearing in the process?

The National Institutes of Health Consensus Development Conference reached some interesting conclusions at their 1990 conference. Here are some of them.

1. Sound levels of less than 75 dB(A) are unlikely to cause permanent hearing loss, while sound levels at 85 dB(A), with exposures of 8 hours per day, will produce permanent hearing loss over a period of ten years or more.

2. More than one third of all hearing losses have occurred (at least in part) from exposure to loud sounds. This means that probably about 2,000,000 people in Canada and about 23,000,000 people in the United States have hearing losses resulting from being exposed to loud noise.

3. Very loud sounds or loud sounds of short duration, such as explosions or gunfire, can produce immediate, severe, and permanent hearing loss. This is called acoustic trauma and instantly damages virtually all the structures in your ears.

4. Longer exposure to less intense, but still hazardous, sounds commonly encountered in the work place or in certain leisure time activities exacts a gradual toll on hearing sensitivity—initially without you being aware of it. Generally, the louder the sound and the longer it lasts—the more severe the resulting hearing loss.

5. About 7 percent of the total population are exposed on a **regular** basis to hazardous noise levels that could result in hearing loss.

The Noise Level Is Too High If . . .

- You need to shout to be heard above the racket.

- Your ears start ringing. This is your ears way of saying "ouch!"

- Voices begin to sound dull or hollow.

- Your ears hurt from the noise.[14]

Being exposed to occupational noise, the most common cause of noise-induced hearing loss, threatens the hearing of fire-fighters, police officers, military personnel, construction and factory workers, musicians, farmers, and truck drivers, to name a few.

Live or recorded high-volume music, whether played back through loud speakers or headphones, is damaging to your ears. This includes the sounds from rock concerts, discotheques and night clubs, personal stereos and the oversized amplifiers in cars and trucks.

Other noisy leisure-time activities include hunting; target practice; skeet shooting; firecrackers; using recreational vehicles such as motorcycles, dirt bikes, speedboats and snowmobiles; flying model airplanes or sitting in the cockpit of private planes; attending car and motorcycle races and other spectator sports; and even playing some video arcade games. Around the house your ears are often exposed to high noise levels when using lawn mowers, snow blowers, chain saws, power tools and some household appliances.

Some medical and dental instruments also produce dangerous noise levels.

6. Noise-induced hearing loss is preventable except in the case of a few accidents. Unfortunately, although it is preventable, our increasingly noisy environment places more and more people at risk of hearing losses.

    It is the acoustic energy of the sound reaching your ears, not its source, which is important. That is, it does not matter if the hazardous sound is generated by a machine in the work place, by a loudspeaker at a rock concert, or by a snowmobile ridden by the listener. Significant amounts of acoustic energy reaching your ears will cause damage—at work, at school, at home, or during leisure activities.

    A .22 calibre rifle can produce a sound of 132 dB per shot. A 12 gauge shotgun is much louder at 172 dB. Did you know that the acoustic energy produced by firing a single round from a shotgun or high-powered rifle is the same as being exposed to a constant noise of 90 dB at work for five 8-hour days? If you fire 50 rounds, you have just caused your ears the same amount of noise damage you would get if you worked in a factory with constant 90 dB noise levels for 1 year![15]

7. Moderate exposure to loud sounds may initially cause a temporary hearing loss. The clinical term for this is a temporary threshold shift (TTS). This is a brief change in hearing that may last for hours or even days. When a TTS occurs, sounds appear to be muffled. Your ears may feel full and may ring or buzz.[16]

Studies have shown that most people attending rock concerts develop a moderate temporary threshold shift. This means that they end up with a hearing loss of about 30 dB as the concert progresses and for a few hours or even a few days after it is over.[17]

With repeated exposure to sounds that cause a TTS or even one severe exposure, your inner ears lose their ability to recover and may gradually cause permanent noise-induced hearing loss. You now have an irreversible permanent threshold shift (PTS).[18] In other words you are now hard of hearing. This can easily happen to you if you attend frequent rock concerts or if you sit too close to the loudspeakers.

8. The first sign of noise-induced hearing loss is usually a loss of sensitivity in the higher frequencies between 3,000 and 6,000 Hz. Your audiogram will typically show a characteristic audiometric "notch." This is because your ears are sensitive to different sounds at different intensities. Certain tones will cause more damage to your ears than others will. Your ears are most sensitive to damage at 4,000 Hz. For example, if you were exposed to a noise composed of all frequencies of sound (white noise) you would first see the typical "noise notch" at 4,000 Hz indicating hearing loss.[19] (Most loud noises are similar to white noise.) With additional hearing loss from noise or aging, the hearing loss at 6,000 and 8,000 Hz may worsen and thus eliminate this characteristic "notch".

9. There is a remarkably broad range of individual differences in sensitivity to any given level of noise. Not all people respond to loud sounds in the

same manner. For example, sounds producing a given hearing loss in one person will likely produce different results in another person. Both temporary and permanent threshold shifts from the same loud noise may differ as much as 30 to 50 dB between people.

10. Hearing conservation must begin by providing each person with basic information about noise and hearing loss. Noise-induced hearing loss is insidious, permanent, and irreparable. It causes communication problems that substantially affect the quality of our lives.

11. Sounds significantly louder than normal speech are potentially harmful if they are present for a sufficient period of time. You can suspect hazardous noise if you experience (a) difficulty communicating while you are exposed to noise, (b) ringing in your ears (tinnitus) after being exposure to loud sounds, and/or (c) muffled hearing after you leave a noisy area.

12. An important consequence of noise-induced hearing loss is difficulty understanding speech. Although a large proportion of the **energy** in speech is contained in the low frequencies, much of the **information** required to differentiate one speech sound from another occurs in the higher frequencies. If you have significant hearing loss in the higher frequencies, you will notice that important speech information is often inaudible or unusable. Other interfering sounds such as background noise, competing voices, room reverberation, and the presence of tinnitus may reduce further your ability to hear.

This noise-induced hearing loss may interfere with your daily life, especially those social activities that occur in noisy settings. It will take more effort to understand speech in these situations. As a result, you will experience more fatigue, anxiety and stress. You will not take part in such activities as often because of this. This will affect not only you, but your family and friends as well and often leads to depression.[20]

13. Noise can make you sick. Studies have shown that noise can quicken your heart rate, increase your blood pressure, and elevate your blood cholesterol levels.[21]

Here's How To Protect Your Ears When Around Noise

As an adult, probably the most important thing you can do to protect your hearing is simply this: don't subject your ears to loud sounds—certainly not for a prolonged time. Remember the effects of noise exposure are long term. They normally don't show up right away. If you expose your ears to continuous loud noise, your ears just wear out faster than normal.

So what should you do if you are around loud noise? If you are free to do so, get out. Simply walk away. You could also turn down the sound level if the volume of a radio, T.V. or stereo is set too high.

If you cannot escape from the noise, keep earplugs handy in your pocket or purse and put them on when the noise level rises. Always wear ear protectors in noisy industrial settings and during noisy hobbies such as hunting and target shooting. Foam rubber ear plugs are good because they are inexpensive, are available over the counter at most drugstores, are not obtrusive and can be quickly rolled up and placed in your ears. They are light, comfortable and easy to carry. Buy ear plugs that have a noise rating of at least 15 dB, preferably higher.[22] Forget about cotton stuffed in your ears—it doesn't give you much protection at all.

The ear muff style of ear protectors give good protection but tend to be more uncomfortable in hot or humid weather. Also, they are considerably more expensive than ear plugs. In spite of this, I like them better and wear them all the time when around loud noises.

Properly fitted ear protectors can reduce sound levels between 15 and 30 dB. Ear plugs are better for protecting your ears from low-frequency noise. Ear muffs work better against high-frequency sounds. Used together, they not only protect your ears from both types of sounds, but give you an additional 10 to 15 dB of protection. In any case, use both together whenever you are around sound levels in excess of 105 dB.[23] Special ear muffs are available for use in excessively noisy conditions. People such as airport workers, jackhammer operators, military personnel and target shooters often wear them. Did you know that many musicians, both classical and rock, wear special custom-made ear plugs during their performances to protect their hearing?[24]

To be effective in protecting your hearing, you must not remove your ear protectors while you are still around noise. Remember, if you are wearing ear protectors with a 30 dB rating and you take them off in a noisy environment, you have just exposed your ears to 1,000 times more sound energy than before.

Incidentally, wearing ear protectors applies to those of us who are hard of hearing as well. Loud sounds will still damage our ears—even though we don't hear them as loud as we once did. Actually, the effects of noise exposure are the same regardless of how loud they seem. Because our little remaining hearing is precious, we do not want to lose any more than we already have lost. Therefore, we must also be careful around loud noises and wear appropriate hearing protection. For example, I always wear ear protectors when using my rototiller, chain saw, hedge clippers, skill saw, table saw, and often when pounding large-sized nails. At the same time, I am amazed how many people with normal hearing do not take such precautions.

If you can't escape the noise, take noise breaks. Your ears need these noise breaks. The longer you expose yourself to loud sounds without a break, the more likely you are to cause permanent damage to your hearing. Therefore, give your ears a 5 or 10 minute break every half hour, even if you are wearing ear plugs.[25]

In your home or office try to reduce the sound level by using sound-absorbing carpets, drapes and upholstered furniture. Place foam pads under (or around) noisy appliances such as food processors and printers. You can help keep the noise level down by only using one noisy appliance at a time. Do not buy toys for your children that produce loud or explosive sounds. Also, before you purchase new appliances, find out how much noise they produce—then buy the quietest model that will do the job.

Noise and Hard of Hearing People— An Intriguing Question

From time to time a hard of hearing person will ask me, "Is the noise damage threshold the same for me as it is for a person with normal hearing? Do I just add my decibel loss (by frequency) to the noise damage threshold for normal ears? If sustained noise at 90 dB is bad for a person with normal hearing, does my noise damage threshold start at 150 dB because I have a 60 dB hearing loss?"

This is an excellent question. I used to wonder about this too. It sounds so plausible on the surface—hard of hearing people can stand far more noise than hearing people. Although this may be true to a **limited** extent for people with conductive hearing losses, it certainly is not true for the vast majority of hard of hearing adults since they have sensorineural hearing losses.

Here is why. Think about this logically. The mechanism of damage is the same whether we have normal hearing or are hard of hearing. Excessively loud sounds permanetly damage our hearing by causing the hair cells containing the minute hairs (cilia) to die. When a hair cell dies, it no longer sends its signal to our brains. As a result we end up with a hearing loss at that frequency of sound.

This would first happen while we still had normal hearing. When enough hair cells die, the message being sent to our brains is not as complete as it once was. But note this—the damage to our inner ears is the same (except now there are fewer hair cells left to die)!

However, if we have a severe or profound loss we may not lose much more hearing from being exposed to loud sounds. This is not because we have a higher tolerance for loud sounds, but because there are not many hair cells left to die! (I've seen pictures where whole banks of hair cells are completely missing. This is quite striking when compared to pictures with all the hair cells there.)

Obviously, the answer to the above question is, "No, you cannot add the amount of your hearing loss to the noise damage threshold to find the amount of noise you can stand without hurting your ears further". It is absolutely false for me to think that since I have a 80 dB loss, I can stand noise at 90 dB plus the 80 dB I am missing for a total of 170 dB before I do any further damage to my hearing.

In fact, I will be writhing in pain long before that ever happens. Why? Remember, most of us with severe or worse losses usually have a severe recruitment problem as well. As a result, our tolerance for loud sounds is actually much **less** than for those with normal hearing. A sound of 110 dB, while very loud to a person with normal hearing may actually give us pain—it may be just too loud for us to stand!

Chapter 3 Endnotes

1   How To Buy A Hearing Aid, 1992. p. 717.
2   Jaret, 1992. pp. 70-71.
3   Vernick, 1993. p. 22
4   Vernick, 1993. p. 146.
5   Huning, 1992. p. 127.
6   Huning, 1992. p. 129.
7   Dudley, 1997. p. 1.
8   Stanten, 1996. p. 13.
9   Staab, 1991. p. 44.
10   Staab, 1991. p. 44.
11   Noise Regulations. 1981.
12   Engel, 1993. pp. 159.
13   Engel, 1993. pp. 159.
14   Staab, 1991. p. 44.
15   Vernick, 1993. p. 148.

16 Vernick, 1993. p. 39.
17 Vernick, 1993. p. 145.
18 Vernick, 1993. p. 40.
19 Vernick, 1993. p. 6.
20 Noise And Hearing Loss, 1990. pp. 1-9.
21 Vernick, 1993. p. 41.
22 Stanten, 1996. pp. 14-15.
23 Vernick, 1993. p. 149.
24 Vernick, 1993. p. 150.
25 Stanten, 1996. p. 15.

Literature Cited

Alpiner, Jerome G. and Patricia A. McCarthy. 1987. Rehabilitative Audiology: Children And Adults. Williams & Wilkins. Baltimore, MD.

Chartrand, Max S. 1988. Psychology Of The Hearing Impaired. Unimax Educational Publications. Texas.

Children and Youth with a Hearing Loss: Promoting Mental Health. 1994. Health Canada. Ottawa, Ontario.

Dudley, John. 1997. Save Your Hearing. jdudley@ worldnet.att.net.

Engel, June. 1993. The Complete Canadian Health Guide. University of Toronto, Faculty of Medicine. Key Porter Books. Toronto, Ontario.

Hardy, Richard E. & John G. Cull. 1974. Educational And Psychosocial Aspects Of Deafness. Charles C Thomas, Publisher. Springfield, Illinois.

Helleberg, Marilyn. 1980. Your Hearing Loss—How To Break The Sound Barrier. Nelson-Hall Inc. Chicago, IL.

Himber, Charlotte. 1989. How To Survive Hearing Loss. G. K. Hall & Co. Thorndike, Maine.

Holt, Judith & Sue Hotto. 1994. Demographic Aspects Of Hearing Impairment: Questions and Answers. Center for Assessment and Demographic Studies. Gallaudet University. Washington, D.C. http://www.gallaudet.edu/~cadsweb/factshee.html.

How To Buy A Hearing Aid. 1992. In: *Consumer Reports.* November, 1992.

Huning, Debbie. 1992. Living Well With Hearing Loss. John Wiley & Sons, Inc. New York.

Ingrao, Bradley B. MS Ed. CCC-A, FAAA, 1996. Hearing and Hearing Loss. Advanced Otolaryngology Services, PA, Jacksonville, FL. http://www.aos-jax.com/h_loss.htm.

Ingrao, Bradley B. 1997. Critical Bands. Personal Communication. Advanced Otolaryngology Services, PA, Jacksonville, FL.

In The Ear Rationale. 1983. Starkey Laboratories, Inc.

Jaret, Peter. 1992. Turn Down The Racket! In: *Readers' Digest.* October, 1992.

Moore, Brian C. 1982. An Introduction To The Psychology of Hearing. Academic Press. London.

New Sounds Inside The Ear. The Daily Telegraph. London. 1989. In: *CHIP Background Information for Speech Reading Instructors.* Extracted from various issues of the British publication, *Catchword.*

Noise And Hearing Loss. 1990. National Institutes of Health Consensus Development Conference Statement. January 22-24, 1990. http://isis.nlm.nih.gov:80/nih/cdc/www/76txt.html.

Noise Regulations, Alberta. AR 3/4/81. Sept. 15, 1981.

Olsson, Robert. 1996. All About Hearing. In: *How-To Guide For Families Coping With Hearing Loss.* http://www.earinfo.com.

Pluvinage, V. 1992. A Review Of ReSound's Technology And Products. ReSound Corporation. Redwood City, CA.

Rezen, Susan & Carl Hausman. 1985. Coping With Hearing Loss: A Guide For Adults And Their Families. Dembner Books. New York, N.Y.

Shimon, Debra. 1992. Coping With Hearing Loss And Hearing Aids. Singular Publishing Group, Inc. San Diego, California.

Staab, Dr. Wayne J. 1991. The Rexton Guide To Better Hearing. 512 East Canterbury Lane, Phoenix, Arizona 85022.

Stanten, Michele. 1996. 150 Secrets To Erase The Signs Of Ageing. Rodale Press, Inc. Emmaus, PA 18098.

Vernick, David M. & Constance Grzelka. 1993. The Hearing Loss Handbook. Consumer Reports Books. Yonkers, N.Y.

Waldhauer, Fred & Edgar Villchur. 1988. Full Dynamic Range Multiband Compression in a Hearing Aid. In: *The Hearing Journal.* Sept. 1988.

Warick, Ruth. 1997. Access for Hard of Hearing Post-Secondary Students—Resource Binder for Service Delivery. Canadian Hard of Hearing Association. Ottawa, ON.

Wilson, Jeanie. 1993. Now Hear This. In: *Readers' Digest.* July, 1993.

Good Books on Hearing Loss

Integrity First Books in the series:

Everything You Wanted to Know About Your Hearing Loss But Were Afraid to Ask (Because You Knew You Wouldn't Hear the Answers Anyway!)

by Neil G. Bauman, Ph.D.

If you have enjoyed this book and would like to learn more about hearing loss and how you can successfully live with it, you may be interested in some helpful books by Dr. Neil. Each book is packed with the things you need to know in order to thrive in spite of your various hearing loss issues. The direct link to the following books is at http://hearinglosshelp.com/shop/category/books/.

Ototoxic Drugs Exposed—The Shocking Truth About Prescription Drugs, Medications, Chemicals and Herbals That Can (and Do) Damage Our Ears
($52.45; eBook $39.95)

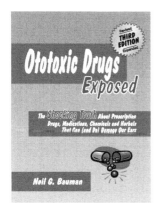

This book, now in its third edition, reveals the shocking truth that many prescription drugs can damage your ears. Some drugs slowly and insidiously rob you of your hearing, cause your ears to ring or destroy your balance. Other drugs can smash your ears in one fell swoop, leaving you with profound, permanent hearing loss and bringing traumatic change into your life. Learn how to protect your ears from the ravages of ototoxic drugs and chemicals. Describes the specific ototoxic effects of 877 drugs, 35 herbals and 148 chemicals (798 pages).

Take Control of Your Tinnitus—Here's How ($29.95; eBook $22.99)

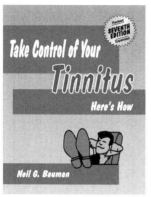

If your ears ring, buzz, chirp, hiss, click or roar, you know just how annoying tinnitus can be. The good news is that you do not have to put up with this racket for the rest of your life. You can take control of your tinnitus. Recent studies show that a lot of what we thought we knew about tinnitus is not true at all. Exciting new research reveals a number of things that you can do to eliminate or greatly reduce the severity of your tinnitus so that it no longer bothers you. This totally-revised, up-to-date and expanded 7th edition contains the very latest in tinnitus research and treatment. In this book you will learn what tinnitus is, what causes tinnitus and things you can do to take control of your tinnitus (356 pages).

Phantom Voices, Ethereal Music & Other Spooky Sounds ($22.49; eBook $16.99)

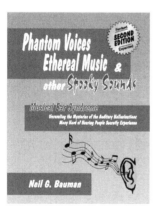

When you realize you are hearing phantom sounds, you immediately think that something has gone dreadfully wrong "upstairs"—that you are going crazy. Because of this, few people openly talk about the strange phantom voices, music, singing and other spooky sounds they hear. This book, the first of its kind in the world, lifts the veil on "Musical Ear syndrome" and reveals numerous first-hand accounts of the many strange phantom sounds people experience. Not only that, it explains what causes these phantom sounds, and more importantly, what you can do to eliminate them, or at least, bring them under control (178 pages).

Say Good Bye to Ménière's Disease—Here's How to Make Your World Stop Spinning ($21.95; eBook $16.49)

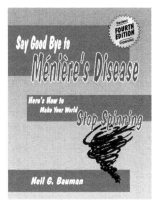

Ménière's disease is one of the more baffling and incapacitating conditions a person can experience. If you suffer from your world spinning, have a fluctuating hearing loss, tinnitus and a feeling of fullness in your ears, this book is for you. It details what Ménière's disease is like; explains the recent breakthrough into the underlying cause of Ménière's; and shows you how, at last, you can be free from the ravages of this debilitating condition. Each page is packed with practical information to help you successfully conquer your Meniere's disease. Join the hundreds and hundreds of people whose worlds have now stopped spinning (128 pages).

Keys to Successfully Living with Your Hearing Loss ($19.97; eBook $15.49)

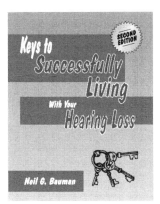

Do you know: a) the critical missing element to successfully living with your hearing loss? b) that the No. 1 coping strategy hard of hearing people instinctively use is wrong, wrong, wrong? c) what the single most effective hearing loss coping strategy is? d) how you can turn your hearing aids into awesome hearing devices? This book addresses the surprising answers to these and other critical questions. Applying them to your life will put you well on the road to successfully living with your hearing loss. (84 pages).

Help! I'm Losing My Hearing—What Do I Do Now? ($18.95; eBook $14.49)

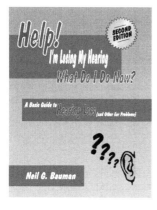

Losing your hearing can flip your world upside down and leave your mind in a turmoil. You may be full of fears, wondering how you will be able to live the rest of your life as a hard of hearing person. You don't know where to turn. You lament, "What do I do now?" Set your mind at rest. This easy to read book, written by a fellow hard of hearing person, is packed with the information and resources you need to successfully deal with your hearing loss and other ear conditions. (116 pages).

Grieving for Your Hearing Loss—The Rocky Road from Denial to Acceptance ($12.95; eBook $9.95)

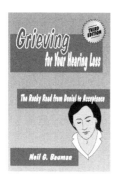

When you lose your hearing you need to grieve. This is not optional—but critical to your continued mental and physical health. This book leads you through the process of dealing with the grief and pain you experience as a result of your hearing loss. It explains what you are going through each step of the way. It gives you hope when you are in the depths of despair and depression. It shows you how you can lead a happy vibrant life again in spite of your hearing loss. This book has helped many (56 pages).

Talking with Hard of Hearing People—Here's How to Do It Right! ($9.95; eBook $7.95)

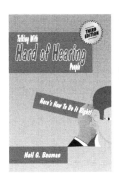

Talking is important to all of us. When communication breaks down, we all suffer. For hard of hearing people this happens all the time. This book is for you—whether you are hearing or hard of hearing! It explains how to communicate with hard of hearing people in one-to-one situations, in groups and meetings, in emergency situations, and in hospitals and nursing homes. When you use the principles given in this book, good things will happen and you will finally be able to have a comfortable chat with a hard of hearing person (38 pages).

When Hearing Loss Ambushes Your Ears—Here's What Happens When Your Hearing Goes on the Fritz ($14.95; eBook $11.95)

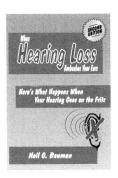

Hearing loss often blind-sides you. As a result, your first step should be to learn as much as you can about your hearing loss; then you will be able to cope better. This most interesting book explains how your ears work, the causes of hearing loss, what you can expect to hear with different levels of hearing loss and why you often can't understand what you hear. Lots of audiograms and charts help make things clear. You will also discover a lot of fascinating things about how loud noises damage your ears (88 pages).

Supersensitive to Sound? You May Have Hyperacusis ($9.95; eBook $7.95)

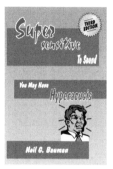

If some (or all) normal sounds seem so loud they blow your socks off, this is the book you want to read! You don't have to avoid noise or lock yourself away in a soundproof room. Exciting new research on this previously baffling problem reveals what you can do to help bring your hyperacusis under control (42 pages).

Here! Here! You and Your Hearing Loss/You and Your Hearing Aids ($12.95; eBook $10.95)

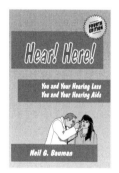

Part I of this book contains a series of my newspaper articles on hearing loss such as, "Hear Today. Gone Tomorrow?" "Hearing Loss Is Sneaky!" "The Wages of Din Is Deaf!" "When Your Ears Ring..." "Get In My Face Before You Speak!" "How's That Again?" "Being Hard of Hearing Is Hard" "I'm Deaf, Not Daft!" Part II contains articles on hearing aids such as, "You Better Watch Out..." "Before Buying Your First Hearing Aid..." "Please Don't Lock Me Away in Your Drawer" "Good-bye World of Silence!" "Becoming Friends with Your Hearing Aids" "Two's Better Than One!" (56 pages).

You can order any of the foregoing books/eBooks
(plus you can read more than 1,000 other helpful
articles about hearing loss and related issues) from the
Center for Hearing Loss Help
web site at
http://hearinglosshelp.com
or order them from the address below

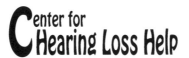

1013 Ridgeway Drive,
Lynden, WA 98264-1057
Phone: (360) 778-1266
FAX: (360) 389-5226
E-mail: info@hearinglosshelp.com
Web site: http://hearinglosshelp.com

Made in the USA
Monee, IL
14 October 2020

44999666R10050